THE GLUCOSE REBELLION

*How I Fired My Pancreas, Rewired My Metabolism,
and Laughed My Way Out of Type 2 Diabetes*

*A Sarcastic, Science-Soaked Survival Guide
for Reversing Type 2 Diabetes and Winning Your Life Back*

By: **Dr. Khalid Saeed, D.O.**

Legal Stuff (Because Lawyers Hate Unregulated Fun)

Medical Disclaimer
The information in this book is for educational, informational, and occasional comedic purposes only. It is **NOT** medical advice, diagnosis, or treatment. Please, please, PLEASE talk to your own doctor before making any major life changes like firing your pancreas, burning your bread stash, or becoming a part-time mitochondria whisperer. Never ignore professional medical advice just because a book made you laugh, cry, and question your breakfast choices. Individual results may vary — because biology is weird.

Author's Disclosure
Dr. Khalid Saeed, D.O., is a licensed physician who has also fought in the trenches of Type 2 diabetes personally. This book is built on a glorious mashup of personal experience, clinical know-how, stubbornness, and entirely too many PubMed articles. Reading this book does **NOT** make me your doctor. (No copays. No waiting rooms. No paperwork. You're welcome.) Consult your own healthcare providers before overhauling your metabolism, staging a glucose rebellion, or doing anything that would make your pancreas do a double take.

Liability Disclaimer
The author and publisher are not liable for any loss, injury, metabolic meltdown, or existential crisis caused by applying the information in this book. Your body, your rebellion, your risk.

Translation: Read responsibly. Laugh liberally. Blame yourself if you eat an entire loaf of banana bread "just to see what happens."

Copyright Notice
© 2025 Khalid Saeed, D.O. / ISBN: 979-8-218-67846-3 / The Glucose Rebellion™
All rights reserved. No part of this book may be reproduced, distributed, or turned into memes without written permission, except for brief quotes used in critical reviews, motivational posters, or sarcastic fridge magnets. Copyright violators will be force-fed cold oatmeal (kidding...mostly).

Trademarks, Satire, Parody, and Commentary Disclaimer
This book contains humorous, satirical, and critical commentary on nutrition science, food marketing, public health guidelines, and widely accepted dietary beliefs. References to processed foods, labeling terms (e.g., "heart-healthy," "low-fat"), branded

dietary advice, and popular nutrition claims are used for educational, nominative, or parody purposes only — not as factual product claims, endorsements, disparagements, or commercial claims. All trademarks remain the property of their respective owners."

All product names, logos, trademarks, and service marks mentioned are the property of their respective owners. Their use in this book is purely **nominative**, for the purposes of **criticism, education, or commentary**, and does **not imply endorsement, affiliation, or approval**.

Any resemblance between fictional metaphors (such as "sugar in a trench coat," "SAD diet," or "glucose crimes") and specific products or brands is purely coincidental. The author's intent is to **critique systemic nutritional misinformation**, not to misrepresent, defame, or malign any individual company or product.

Humor is used throughout to **demystify complex health topics** and promote behavior change through accessibility and engagement. Satire and parody are **protected forms of expression** under U.S. copyright law (17 U.S.C. §107) and reinforced by case law such as *Campbell v. Acuff-Rose Music*, 510 U.S. 569 (1994).

All illustrations are a work of satire and parody, created for **educational and humorous** purposes. Any resemblance to specific brands, products, or franchises (such as light swords or snack packaging) is purely coincidental and not intended to imply affiliation, endorsement, or ownership. All characters are fictional, and this artwork is protected under fair use (17 U.S.C. §107) as transformative commentary.

If your feelings are hurt by jokes about cereal boxes, granola bars, or quinoa marketing, please note: this book is not intended to defame, mislead, or maliciously target any person or product. It's meant to make you **laugh, think, and maybe question your pantry**.

If you're unsure whether you were personally insulted, or your breakfast cereal was, or your endocrinologist was… you probably just need a snack.

Credits
Cover design, interior layout, and illustrations by Khalid Saeed, D.O.

DEDICATION

For everyone who ever trusted a food label. For every pancreas that waved the white flag while we spooned "healthy" oatmeal into our mouths. For the mitochondria that kept trying, even when we didn't deserve it. And for anyone who's ever looked at a Continuous Glucose Monitor (CGM) graph and thought, *"Well, that escalated quickly."* This rebellion is for you.

"The best way to predict your future is to stop outsourcing it to the empire of edible lies hiding behind kid-friendly branding and adult-sized consequences."

— Technically accurate advice. Now fortified with sarcasm, science, and a sprinkle of rebellion.

ACKNOWLEDGMENTS

To the scientists who said, "Maybe the food pyramid is, in fact, a pyramid scheme."

To the patients who trusted me — especially when I became the patient myself.

To my family and friends who endured spontaneous glucose lectures, guacamole evangelism, and suspiciously passionate arguments about cauliflower rice.

To my CGM for snitching on my bread addiction and saving my pancreas.

To the editors, researchers, mentors, and adrenaline — without whom this book would just be a series of unhinged rants typed at 3 AM.

And to humor — for turning glucose graphs, metabolic crashes, and pantry purges into punchlines instead of prison sentences.

Without you, this book would just be science.

With you, it became survival, rebellion, and a whole lot of sarcastic hope.

TABLE OF CONTENTS

Dedication i
Acknowledgments iii

Introduction: I Diagnosed Myself... Then Fired My Pancreas 1
Part I: Diagnosis Drama 5
Chapter 1: So Your Pancreas Is On Strike 7
Chapter 2: Bread Is a Liar and Other Metabolic Truth Bombs 11
Chapter 3: Habits Are Hard. Science Helps 17

Part II: Battle Plan for Metabolic Rebellion 23
Chapter 4: Grocery Shopping Like a Glucose Master 25
Chapter 5: Kitchen Makeover: Diabetic Edition 29
Chapter 6: Recipes That Won't Spike Your Meter or Bore Your Soul .. 33
Chapter 7: Exercise — Move It or Lose It (To Insulin Resistance) 37
Chapter 8: Glucose Monitoring — The Feedback Loop That Shames Your Meal Choices 43

Part III: Leveling Up Your Comeback Story 49
Chapter 9: Surviving Real Life — Cravings, Parties, and Plateau Purgatory 51
Chapter 10: This Isn't a Diet — It's a Comeback Story 55
Chapter 11: Meds, Myths, and Metabolic Middlemen 59
Chapter 12: Resources for Nerds, Newbies, and Everyone in Between 63

Bonus Level 69
Bonus Chapter: Intermittent Fasting — Your Metabolic Cheat Code . 71
Conclusion: Welcome to the Rest of Your Life 77

About The Author 81
References 83
Suggested Reading 85
Glossary of Terms 89

INTRODUCTION:
I DIAGNOSED MYSELF...
THEN FIRED MY PANCREAS

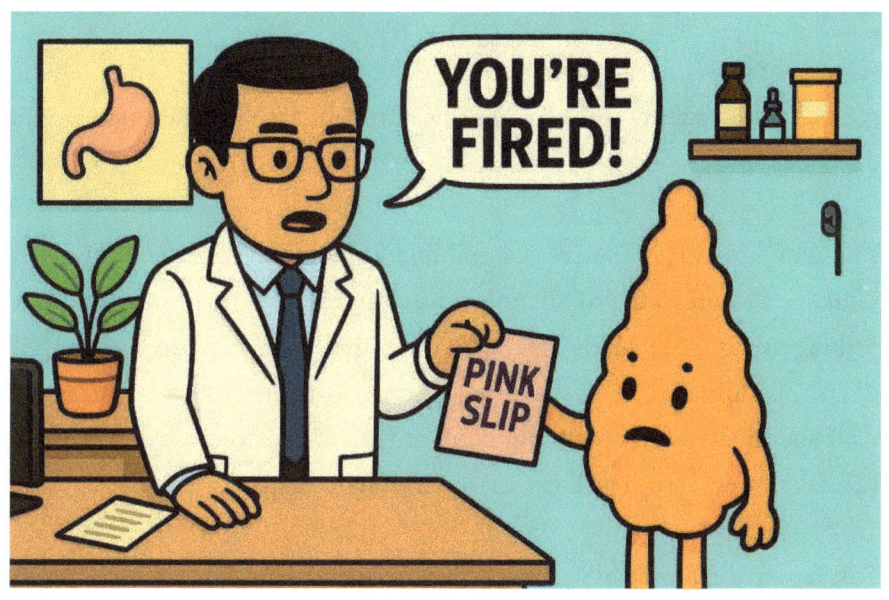

Imagine *the scene: There I am—a fully licensed, board-certified physician, trained to detect diseases at fifty paces. My brain? Razor-sharp. My pantry? A metabolic crime scene. I was dispensing life-saving advice by day...and personally keeping the cereal industry afloat by night.*

Cue the biochemical betrayal: My A1c strolls in at a blazing 8.6% (For reference, normal is below 5.7%. Anything 6.5% and up? That's full-blown diabetes territory.). Energy levels? Missing, presumed dead. Bathroom trips? Frequent enough to qualify for loyalty points. Waistline? Declared itself a sovereign nation—complete with borders, a flag, and a

GDP made entirely of refined carbohydrates. Bonus: blurry vision and enough dizziness to qualify as a theme park ride.

Plot twist: I became the patient. Yes, a doctor who knew exactly what insulin resistance was...and now needed a mirror pep talk just to explain it to himself. Cue existential crisis. Cue professional irony.

Instead of surrendering to a future filled with pill organizers and diabetic socks, I did what any stubborn, nerdy, adrenaline-charged human would do:

I fired my exhausted pancreas. I grabbed a glucometer and a Continuous Glucose Monitor (CGM) like they were endocrine disruptor detectors. I binge-read PubMed like it was the last season of CSI: Metabolism, and the finale was coming for my A1c. I unleashed Carbageddon on my pantry and nuked it into a no-carb wasteland. I turned myself into a walking, low-carb science experiment.

Fast forward 10 months:
- 80 pounds? Gone.
- Blood sugar? Normalized.
- Medications? Never started.
- Sanity? Barely intact, but totally worth it.

What I Found (Hint: It Wasn't In the Nutrition Guidelines)

Type 2 diabetes isn't just about blood sugar. It's about insulin resistance — and a system that's been quietly failing for years before the glucose carnage shows up.

It's not just "genetics" or "willpower." It's chronic exposure to a food supply engineered to break your metabolism and a culture that tells you it's your fault when it does.

The good news? Insulin resistance is reversible. Even better news? You don't need 12 medications, 6 specialists, or a second mortgage to pull it off. Best news? You can fix it with science, systems, stubbornness, and a little (okay, a lot of) sarcasm.

What This Book Is

A lovechild of **clinical science** *(because feelings aren't biomarkers).*

Real-world self-experimentation *(with side effects like hope, curiosity, and a lot of guacamole).*

Weaponized humor *(because sarcasm won't lower insulin...but it will make you embrace broccoli without sobbing).*

This isn't a diet guide. It's a **full-scale, evidence-based rebellion**. It's a **comeback story** — powered by mitochondria, memes, and mild amounts of rage.

If you're here because you're tired of diabetes bossing you around... welcome, friend. This is your **Metabolic Reboot Manual**. Grab your lab coat and your sass — it's time to stage your own Glucose Rebellion.

Why This Book Exists

Because the world doesn't need another boring diabetes manual full of sad food pyramids and "everything in moderation" lies. It needs a rebellion.

This book is the survival guide I wish I had when I first watched my CGM graph go full rollercoaster after "whole-grain halo-wearing" oatmeal.

It's for anyone who's ever: Been blindsided by a diagnosis they didn't see coming. Felt trapped by a body that refuses to cooperate. Questioned if there was a better way. Wanted to fight back without giving up coffee, joy, and the will to live.

How This Book Works

Short chapters. Tactical advice. Just enough science. Light ego. Side servings of sarcasm when necessary (always). Zero toxic positivity. Zero shame spirals.

You'll learn: How your metabolism actually works (and how it got hijacked). How carbs aren't evil — but they are often double agents. How insulin became a hormonal drama queen. How to shop, cook, move, fast, and live like your mitochondria are finally in charge. How to rebuild from scratch — without hating your life.

Fair Warning

This isn't a diet book. This isn't a magic bullet. This isn't going to tell you to "cut fat, not carbs"—because that worked so well the first time.

This is a blueprint for taking back control — with science, humor, and zero patience for Glucose Denial Syndrome.

If you're ready to laugh, learn, and launch an uprising inside your own mitochondria...Let's go.

Welcome to **The Glucose Rebellion**™.

PART I:
DIAGNOSIS DRAMA

CHAPTER 1:
SO YOUR PANCREAS IS ON STRIKE

When Your Glucose Thinks It's the Main Character.

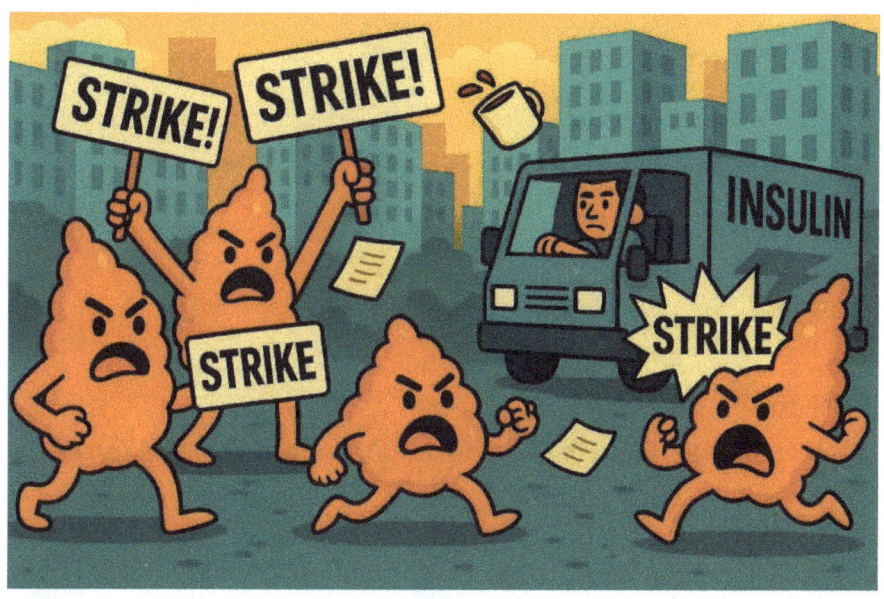

Let's paint you a beautiful, horrifying picture. Imagine your body as a bustling metropolis:

- **Glucose** = the electricity keeping the city lit.
- **Insulin** = the truck drivers delivering the energy.
- **Your Cells** = the homes and buildings waiting for packages like hormonal porch pirates.

In a healthy setup?
- Glucose flows.
- Insulin delivers.
- The city shines.

*In **Type 2 diabetes**?*
- The houses slap up a neon "NO DELIVERIES" sign.
- The insulin trucks pile up like abandoned scooters downtown.
- Traffic jams erupt.
- Your poor, overworked **pancreas** is screaming into the void, furiously dispatching *more* insulin trucks, while the cells are out back vaping and ghosting deliveries.

*Eventually, the pancreas — underpaid, overworked, and drowning in carbs it didn't approve — slams its clipboard down, flips over the metabolic table, and **goes on strike**. — "I'm Out!"*

Welcome to your biochemical dumpster fire.

Translation Station:

If you prefer your biochemistry without the screaming metaphors:

Term	Reality Check
Insulin Resistance	Your cells ghost insulin harder than your worst blind date.
Hyperinsulinemia	Your pancreas is panic-texting insulin into the bloodstream: rapid, unfiltered, and way too much.
Type 2 Diabetes	A full-scale cellular mutiny. Bad for vibes. Worse for organs.

How To Annoy Your Pancreas Into Quitting:

(Or: How Modern Life Played You)

- **Genetics:** A family recipe for sarcasm, shaky mitochondria, and a fruit-triggered metabolic alarm system.

- **Chronic Stress:** Modern life is basically one long cortisol kegger.
- **Sleep Deprivation:** Nothing screams "future metabolic disaster" like binge-watching streaming shows until your eyeballs are dry.
- **Standard American Diet (SAD):** If edible oil products, high fructose corn syrup, and nutritional propaganda had a baby, it would be called the SAD diet.

Science Snapshot:

"**Visceral fat — especially around the liver and pancreas — drives insulin resistance by fueling chronic inflammation and mitochondrial dysfunction.**"

— *Taylor et al., Diabetologia, 2012*

Translation: *That "dad bod" isn't just a fashion statement. It's an inflammatory cytokine-spewing factory whispering lies into your pancreas's ear like some biochemical Mean Girl: "Pssst... Don't trust insulin. He's totally fake."*

The Good News (Yes, There's Hope):

Type 2 diabetes is not a final boss.
It's more like an annoying mini-boss you can body-slam with science, stubbornness, and a better grocery list.

It's not *cured* — we're not handing out fairy tale endings — but **reversed**, like blocking a toxic ex on all social media and finally moving on.

It's not your fault. It's your system.

Systems can crash. Systems can reboot. And you, my friend, are about to stage the sassiest, science-iest reboot this side of endocrinology.

Doctor's Orders (Now With Extra Snark):

- **Stop blaming yourself.** Your pancreas isn't mad at you. It's mad at a thousand tiny systemic insults.
- **Get curious, not judgmental.** Your metabolism isn't a moral failing. It's a pissed-off biochemical symphony.
- **Understand fuel quality.** Not all carbs are evil. But a lot of them are dressed like wellness influencers while secretly plotting your downfall.
- **New goal:** Lower your insulin load. Build muscle. Stabilize glucose. — **Bonus goal:** Beat your pancreas at its own overdramatic game.

Final Snarky Mic Drop:

Type 2 diabetes isn't a personality trait.

It's a system error — and systems can be rebuilt. Preferably with protein, fiber, good memes, and the occasional side-eye at anything labeled "heart healthy" in the cereal aisle.

CHAPTER 2:
BREAD IS A LIAR AND OTHER METABOLIC TRUTH BOMBS

How Your "Healthy" Oatmeal Committed Biochemical Treason

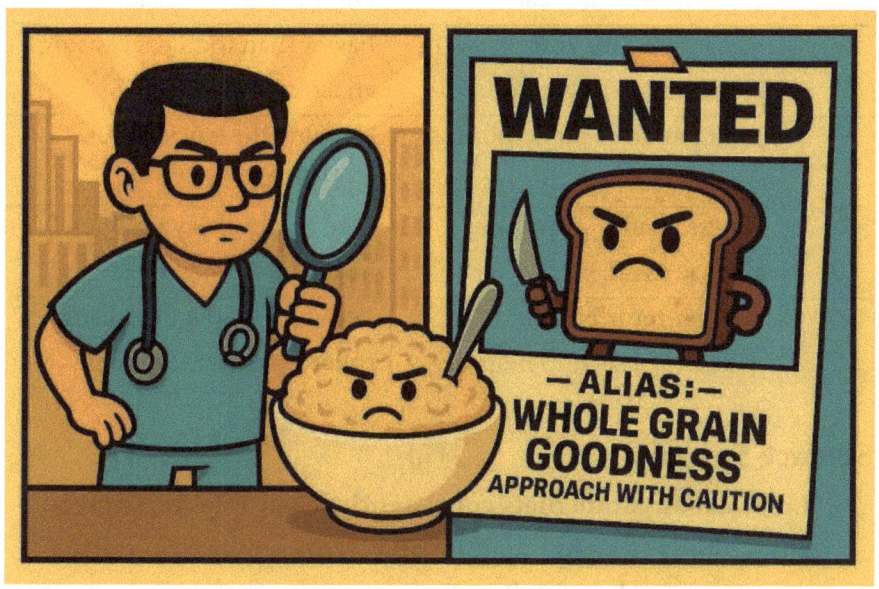

Raise your hand if you've ever been personally victimized by a "Whole Grain Goodness!" label. *(Raises both hands, a foot, and a skeptical eyebrow.)*

Picture it: I'm building the Pinterest-perfect breakfast — organic oatmeal, ethically sourced berries, virtuous flaxseed sprinkled like fairy dust.

Cue the Continuous Glucose Monitor (CGM): The graph spiked so hard it filed a police report.

Plot twist: That "nutritious" oatmeal? Just sugar in a fiber trench coat trying to sneak past your pancreas.

The Great Carb Conspiracy:

Let's untangle the glucose con game:

Step	What Happens	Why It's Sketchy
1	You eat "healthy" carbs.	Oatmeal, quinoa, sadness.
2	They slam into your bloodstream as glucose.	Faster than toddlers chasing an ice cream truck.
3	Your pancreas panic-dumps insulin.	"Deploy the trucks! ALL THE TRUCKS!"
4	Excess insulin stores the glucose as fat.	Like a doomsday prepper hoarding canned beans.
5	Hunger returns faster than guilt after a second helping.	Welcome to the blood sugar rollercoaster of doom.

Science Snapshot:

> "Low-carbohydrate diets consistently lower HbA1c, triglycerides, body weight, and insulin requirements — often outperforming low-fat diets."
>
> — *Saslow et al., Nutrition, 2017*

Translation: Low-carb isn't a fad. It's **metabolic rehab** with protein as your emotional support animal.

"Healthy Carbs" Are Basically Double Agents:

- **Oatmeal?** Raises your blood sugar almost as much as straight-up table sugar in a lab study.
- **"Whole wheat" bread?** Sends your glucose higher than white bread half the time. (Glycemic impact: unpredictable at best.)

- **Brown rice?** Less evil than candy, but still holding hands with insulin resistance at a molecular level.

Carb Math 101:

Fewer carbs → Less insulin → Less fat storage → Less "I hate my pants."

Diet Style	Daily Carb Limit	Nickname
Moderate Carb	<130g	"Still-Sorta-Sugary"
Low Carb	<100g	"Smart Carb"
Keto	<50g	"Serious About Science"
Dr. Saeed's Happy Place	30–50g	"Insulin Zen Zone"

What Actually Worked For Me (Aka: Metabolic Master Training)

Stopped calorie-counting. Because your mitochondria don't care about math — they care about substrate quality.

Stopped fearing fat. Turns out, avocados aren't plotting your death. (I'm looking at you, 1990's nutrition guidelines.)

Stopped eating snack bars made of granola, high-fructose sadness, and food pyramid propaganda.

Instead, I rebuilt every meal around the holy trinity: **Protein + Fiber + Fat** = The Hunger Busting Dream Team.

How Cutting Carbs Unfroze My Metabolism:

- Blood glucose calmed down.
- Insulin stopped behaving like an unhinged toddler at a birthday party.
- Fat storage slowed down, then reversed.
- Inflammation packed its cytokine suitcases and left.
- Insulin sensitivity staged a heroic comeback montage.

Bonus: My suits and I became friends again after years of silent resentment.

Smart Swaps (Because You Still Deserve Joy)

Instead of…	Fuel Up With…
Whole grain crackers	Cheese crisps or cucumber slices
Bananas	Berries (the MVP of low-glycemic fruits)
Rice	Cauliflower rice (surprisingly magical)
Pasta	Zoodles (spiralized zucchini, not sadness)

Pro Tip: Cauliflower rice might smell weird while cooking, but it won't assassinate your glucose.

Bonus Nerd Stuff: Morning Carbs Hit Harder (Here's Why)

Your body is naturally more insulin resistant in the morning — a fun, circadian gift from your liver and adrenal glands. Thanks to the **dawn**

phenomenon, cortisol and growth hormone spike in the early hours to help you wake up, but they also raise your blood sugar and make your cells **less responsive** to insulin.

Translation? That same bowl of oatmeal will spike your glucose like a rocket at 8 AM, but might barely budge it at 6 PM.

Science Snapshot:

> **"Identical meals eaten at breakfast triggered significantly higher glucose and insulin spikes than when eaten at dinner — proving that your morning metabolism is basically still asleep."**
>
> — *Jakubowicz et al., Diabetologia, 2015*

Translation: Your cells aren't morning people. Eat your carbs later, or get ready for a blood sugar rollercoaster before your coffee even kicks in.

Why It Happens:

Blame your circadian rhythm — the body's internal clock that controls everything from hormone release to metabolic readiness. In the early morning, your cortisol and growth hormone levels are naturally higher (to help wake you up), but they also **increase insulin resistance**.

Your liver, meanwhile, thinks it's being helpful by dumping extra glucose into your bloodstream — just in case you need to wrestle a bear before breakfast. The result? More glucose + more resistance = a hormonal traffic jam.

Translation:

Your body's like, "Here's some sugar for survival!"

Your cells are like, "Not now, bro, I'm still booting up."

The fix: Keep breakfast lower in carbs and higher in **protein + healthy fats** to smooth out the morning glucose chaos. Think: eggs and avocado instead of toast and jam. Save the carbs (if you eat them at all) for later in the day, when your cells are a bit more cooperative.

Final Snarky Mic Drop:

*This isn't about carb-phobia. It's about **metabolic justice.***

It's not about punishment. It's about **taking back biochemical control** from sneaky oatmeal assassins.

New motto for life: **"Bread lies. Science rides."**

CHAPTER 3:
HABITS ARE HARD. SCIENCE HELPS

Why Willpower Is a Scam and Systems Are Your Survival Gear

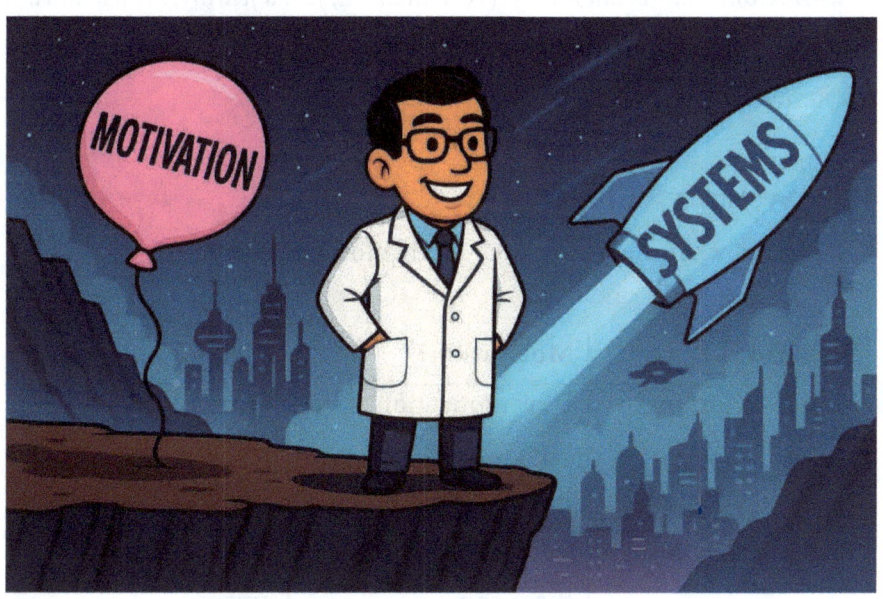

Here's some straight talk: **Willpower is a garbage business model.**

It's like investing in floppy disks in 2025. It *might* work for about 20 minutes on a Monday morning…but by Thursday at 4:59 PM, you're talking to a vending machine like a hostage negotiator with Stockholm syndrome.

If success required constant motivation, I would still be sitting on the couch mainlining granola bars and blaming "bad genetics."

Motivation *feels good*. Systems **actually work**.

Science Snapshot:

"You do not rise to the level of your goals. You fall to the level of your systems."

— *James Clear, Atomic Habits*

Translation: Your brain is lazy. (Not an insult, just a feature.) It will always default to whatever's easiest. You either **build easy GOOD defaults**, or you live in snack regret purgatory forever.

Why Systems > Vibes:

Systems are what catch you when motivation face-plants.

Scenario	Motivation?	Systems?
Monday Morning	Peak motivation ("New week, new me!")	Same
Thursday Night	Zero left ("I deserve these chips.")	System triggers anyway
Aunt Linda's Birthday	Cake is singing siren songs	Preloaded plan saves you
Existential crisis at 11 PM	Motivation buried under online streaming guilt	System drags you to safety

The Science Of System Hacking:

Here's how I rebuilt my metabolism, my wardrobe, and my will to live — without trusting my sad, weak-willed human nature:

Habit	Why It Worked	Science Flex
<50g carbs/day	Slashed insulin demand like a metabolic ninja	Lower glucose = lower hunger = lower drama
Target A1c <5.5%	Gave me a scoreboard to obsess over	Metrics > Feelings
Daily 20-min walks	Increased insulin sensitivity	Moving muscles = glucose disposal VIP pass
Tiny plates for meals	Tricked my brain into feeling full	Visual illusions are your frenemy
Prioritized PFF (Protein + Fiber + Fat)	Kept blood sugar flatter than a pancake	Stabilized glucose, nuked cravings

Instead of…	Choose This…	Why?
Potato chips	Roasted almonds, cheese crisps	Fat + salt = satisfaction without glucose carnage
Candy bars	85% dark chocolate (the emo poet of sweets)	Low sugar, high smugness
Granola	Chia seed pudding (fiber grenade)	Keeps hunger locked up like Fort Knox
Oatmeal	Greek yogurt + berries	Real food > glucose fireworks

Smarter, Sassier Swaps:
Habit Hacks For Metabolic Rebels:

Stack it: Attach new habits to existing ones.
"After brushing my teeth → check my CGM."

Track it: You can't manage what you're pretending not to see. (Spoiler: Hope is NOT a strategy.)

Forgive it: One carb crime is not a felony.
Log it. Laugh at it. Walk it off. Plot your revenge against bread later. It's best served cold anyway. (The revenge, not the bread.)

Science Snapshot:

"Habit formation, self-monitoring, and consistent meal planning are associated with superior metabolic control and weight maintenance."
— *Wing et al., NEJM, 2001; Hall et al., Nutrition Reviews, 2019*

Translation: *Hope is cute. Data is undefeated.*

True Story:

(Prepare for some relatable failure)

My first week?

- Too tired (ie. lazy) to walk.
- Stress-ate an entire sleeve of cookies.
- CGM graph looked like the stock market crash of 1929.

Did I cry? Maybe. Did I quit? No. Did I log it, laugh at it, and keep moving like the petty, stubborn mitochondria maverick I am? **Absolutely.** Ten months later, my pancreas sends me metaphorical thank-you notes.

Mantra For The Metabolic Rebellion:
"Consistency beats intensity. Every. Single. Time."

Forget "perfect." Forget "motivated." Focus on "still showing up" — even when you don't feel like it. That's where metabolic magic actually happens.

PART II:
BATTLE PLAN FOR METABOLIC REBELLION

CHAPTER 4:
GROCERY SHOPPING LIKE A GLUCOSE MASTER

*How to Dodge Cereal Lies and Shop
Like Your Metabolism Depends on It — Because It Absolutely Does*

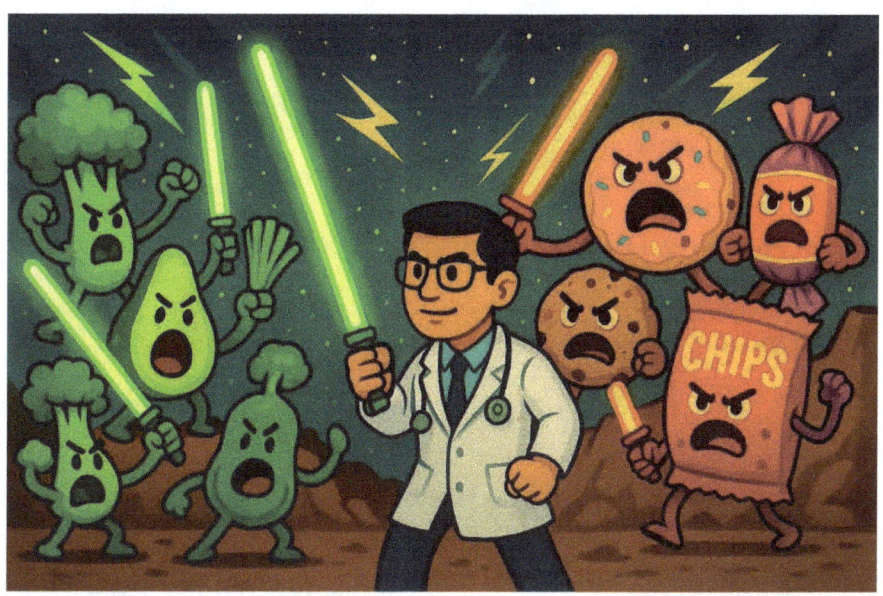

Here's a fun fact they never tell you: **Grocery stores are biochemical ambush zones.**

Bright lights. Strategic shelf placement. Entire aisles of glucose bombs dressed up as nutritious heroes. It's not a grocery run — it's **Pancreas Games: Metabolic Edition.**

But you? You're about to become a **Glucose Master**. Laser sword optional. Label-decoding mandatory.

The Glucose Master Grocery Code:

- *Shop the Perimeter:* Vegetables, meats, eggs, dairy. That's where real food lives. Middle aisles? That's where "food-like substances" plot your metabolic downfall.
- *Distrust Health Halos:* If the box screams about how healthy it is, it's lying louder than a bad online dating profile.
- *Flip the Box:* Never trust the front. Read the back label like it owes you money.
- *Beware Sneaky Words:* Always look for the hidden sugars. If it ends in "-ose" (glucose, fructose, maltose) —Translation: Sugar, sugar, sugar, betrayal.

Label Reading 101: Metabolic Detective Mode

Label Trap	Why It's Trash
"Net carbs"	Fiber math sorcery designed to fool your pancreas.
"Organic cane sugar"	Still sugar. Now just smug about it.
"Agave nectar"	Blood sugar betrayal in syrup form.
"Multigrain"	Multiplied your glucose spike. Congratulations.

Golden Rule: If it sounds like a super villain or an alchemy ingredient, don't eat it.

Build A Sane Plate (Visualize It Like A Battle Plan):

Section	Food Type	Mission
½ Plate	Non-starchy vegetables	Micronutrient armor
¼ Plate	Protein (chicken, fish, beef)	Muscle fuel + satiety bomb
¼ Plate	Healthy fats (avocado, olive oil, nuts)	Hormone optimization & flavor joy

Goal: Every meal = biochemical ceasefire between you and your mitochondria.

Science Snapshot:

"Meal preparation, strategic shopping, and a healthy home food environment are strongly associated with improved glycemic control and weight outcomes."

— Gudzune et al., Obesity Research, 2015

Translation: Buy garbage = eat garbage = feel like garbage. Stock real food = eat real food = metabolically flex on your enemies.

Grocery Store Survival Hacks:

- **Never shop hungry:** If you're already fantasizing about double chocolate chunk cookies, turn the car around.
- **Make a list:** Treat it like a Navy SEAL mission dossier. Free-styling = snack aisle disaster.
- **Stick to the list:** If you wander, so will your insulin.
- **Avoid the carb ambush aisles:** ("Breakfast foods," "Snack foods," "Betrayal foods.")
- **Bring a smug reusable grocery bag:** Intimidate the processed foods into submission.

Death Traps To Avoid:

Aisle	Ambush
Breakfast	97% sugar in a costume
Snacks	"Organic kale puffs" still spike glucose
Drinks	If it's not water, tea, or coffee, it's sugar with a PR agent
Baking	Where dreams — and blood sugar stability — go to die

Warning: The "healthy snack" aisle is just a sugar trap with better branding.

Stock Your Pantry Like A Metabolic Warlord:

Category	Must-Haves
Proteins	Eggs, steak, salmon, Greek yogurt, sardines (if you're brave)
Healthy Fats	Avocados, olive oil, butter (yes, butter)
Vegetables	Broccoli, spinach, zucchini, cauliflower
Smart Swaps	Almond flour, coconut flour, miracle noodles
Snacks	Roasted almonds, cheese crisps, 85% dark chocolate (the broody poet of sweets)

Wisdom: If your kitchen whispers *"We stabilize glucose here,"* you're winning. If it whispers *"We have frosted brownies hidden behind the quinoa,"* you're doomed.

Final Snarky Mic Drop:

A battle-ready grocery cart beats heroic willpower every single time. You don't fight insulin resistance with good vibes and desperate prayers. You fight it with pre-loaded vegetables, fatty acids, protein bombs, and a ruthless disrespect for the cereal aisle.

CHAPTER 5:
KITCHEN MAKEOVER: DIABETIC EDITION

Extreme Homeostasis — Purging Your Pantry Like Your Life Depends on It, Because It Does

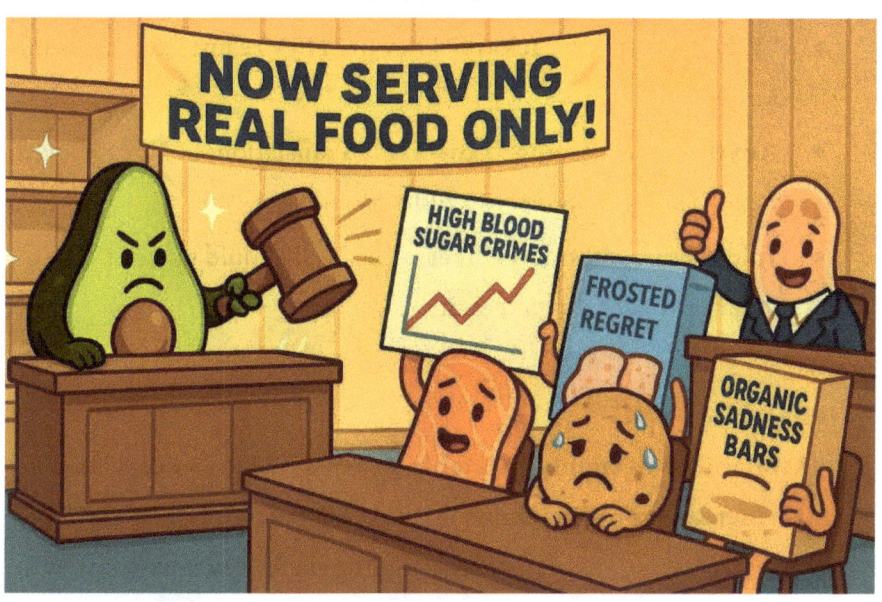

CUE the cold, hard truth: **You can't out-walk, out-pray, or out-supplement a pantry full of Sugary Snacks and broken dreams.**

Your kitchen is either your ally or your assassin.

If your cabinets look like a sugar bomb went off in a supermarket clearance aisle: Congratulations — you're making diabetes the landlord of your metabolism.

29

Time to evict the junk food. Ruthlessly. Without mercy. Even if you have to take it to court.

Step One: Purge Like A Savage

- ***Cereal:*** *Dessert pretending to be breakfast. Even the ones with cheerful cartoon critters are guilty.*
- **Granola Bars:** Candy bars with gym memberships.
- **Pasta:** Long, stringy insulin spikes.
- **"Whole Grain" Crackers:** They lie. They're just salsa chips in khaki pants.
- **Anything Screaming "Low-Fat":** Translation — *"We removed fat, added sugar, and now it tastes like sadness."*
- **Juice:** Fruit without the fiber — basically liquid glucose with a vitamin sticker slapped on it.

Science Snapshot:

"Availability of highly palatable processed foods correlates with increased energy intake, insulin resistance, and obesity."
— Lustig et al., *Metabolical,* 2021

Translation: *Your kitchen is quietly staging a coup against your pancreas if you don't take control.*

Step Two: Restock For Metabolic Domination

Category	Load Up On	Mission
Proteins	Eggs, steak, chicken, fish, Greek yogurt	Muscle fuel + satiety overlords
Healthy Fats	Avocados, olive oil, butter	Hormone whisperers
Low-Starch Veggies	Broccoli, spinach, zucchini, cauliflower	Micronutrient ninjas
Smart Swaps	Almond flour, coconut flour, miracle noodles	Lower carbs, higher metabolic flex

Golden Rule: If your new pantry doesn't whisper "Mitochondrial Gala," you're not done yet.

Step Three: Kitchen Gadgets Of Glucose Domination

- **Cast Iron Skillet:** Because our ancestors didn't sear steaks on non-stick pans. Be legendary.
- **Veggie Spiralizer:** Turns zucchini into zoodles — and regret into hope.
- **Mini Food Scale:** Because "eyeballing portions" is how "just one handful of nuts" becomes "1,200 accidental calories."
- **Continuous Glucose Monitor (CGM):** Truth serum for your meal choices. CGM graphs: now with 100% less denial.

Kitchen Setup = Your Secret Weapon:

If you...	You Will...
Pre-chop veggies	Actually eat them
Hard-boil eggs weekly	Beat cravings at 4 PM without caving
Portion snacks ahead of time	Avoid "handful inflation" syndrome
Keep tempting junk out of sight (or house)	Save your pancreas unnecessary betrayal

Pro tip: Out of sight = out of mouth. If you have to climb a ladder, open three boxes, and fight off a dust bunny just to find a cookie... You'll eat the roasted chicken instead.

Science Snapshot:

"**Structured home food environments strongly predict adherence to healthy eating behaviors and improved metabolic outcomes.**"

— Gorin et al., Obesity Research, 2005

Translation: Your environment wins every argument your willpower loses. Set it up like you mean it.

Final Snarky Mic Drop:

You are not "bad at diets." You are "bad at surviving in an environment engineered to make you metabolically implode." Fix your environment = Fix your odds. No shame. No drama. Just biochemical reality. Your kitchen isn't just a room. **It's your metabolic command center.** *Equip it like a rebel base. Not like a hostage negotiation van.*

CHAPTER 6:
RECIPES THAT WON'T SPIKE YOUR METER OR BORE YOUR SOUL

Meals That Taste Like Freedom, Not Hospital Cafeteria Regret

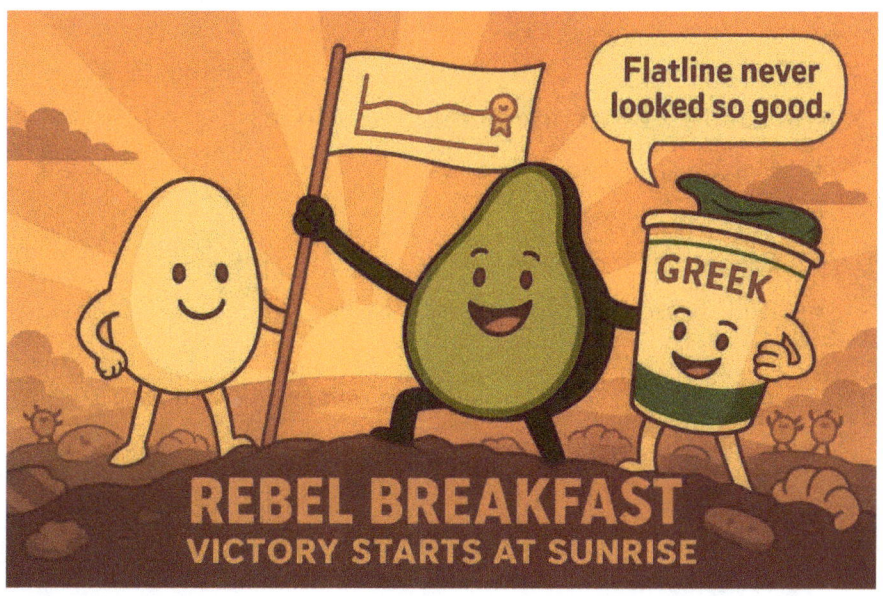

Let's kill a myth right now: **Low-carb eating does not mean surviving on boiled chicken, kale tears, and existential dread.**

You are not being sentenced to culinary purgatory. You are **being liberated** from blood sugar whiplash disguised as "whole grain goodness." You deserve meals that: Stabilize your glucose. Taste like you still love life. Don't require a PhD in Molecular Gastronomy.

Breakfast: Declaration Of Pancreatic Peace
1. Spinach Omelet of Champions
- 2 eggs
- Handful of spinach
- Pinch of feta cheese
- Salsa if you're feeling frisky

Outcome: Fast. Delicious. Blood sugar stays flatter than your last bad haircut.

2. Avocado Egg Bowl (Metabolic Flex Mode)
- Halve an avocado.
- Crack an egg inside.
- Bake at 375°F for ~15 minutes.
- Add cheese and seasoning because you deserve happiness.

Translation: You're telling your mitochondria, "I respect you now"

3. Greek Yogurt Redemption Parfait
- Full-fat, unsweetened Greek yogurt
- ¼ cup berries
- Sprinkle of cinnamon because metabolic flair matters
- Optional: DIY chia seed granola for extra fiber flex

Warning: You may accidentally Instagram this. No judgment.

Lunch & Dinner: Blood Sugar Redemption Arc
1. Chicken Power Bowl (Lunchroom Mic Drop)
- Base: Cabbage or kale
- Protein: Grilled chicken
- Extras: Avocado, cucumber, tahini drizzle

Mission: *Stabilize insulin. Crush cravings. Leave hunger sobbing in the corner.*

2. Cauliflower Fried Rice (Ninja-Level Trickery)
- Blitz cauliflower into "rice."
- Sauté with eggs, scallions, coconut aminos.
- Add leftover steak or shrimp because you're smart.

Pro Tip: *Use chopsticks. Feels fancy. Burns more calories. (Probably.)*

3. Roasted Salmon + Veggie Squad
- Salmon + olive oil + herbs
- Brussels sprouts roasted till crispy

Bonus: *Omega-3s = Anti-inflammatory superpowers. Also = Smug health superiority.*

4. Bunless Burger with Dignity
- Beef patty in a lettuce wrap (or between two roasted portobellos)
- Add cheese, mustard, sarcasm

Optional Side Dish: *Eye-roll at fast food commercials.*

Snacks: Pancreas-Friendly Damage Control
- ***Deviled Eggs:*** *Fatty, filling, gourmet if you squint hard enough.*
- **Fat Bombs:** Coconut oil + almond butter + cocoa = edible joy grenades.
- **85% Dark Chocolate:** One square = maximum vibes, minimum spike.
- **Cheese Crisps:** Crunchy rebellion against glucose tyranny.

Science Snapshot:

"Low glycemic-load meals improve satiety, prevent post-prandial glucose excursions, and reduce rebound hunger."

— Ludwig et al., JAMA, 2002

Translation: Eat smart. Stay full. Stop chasing snacks like a rabid raccoon at 3 PM.

Pro Cooking Tip:

*If your meals are: Colorful, full of actual nutrients, satisfying enough to make you hum happily while eating...***You're winning.** *(Also, you're making your pancreas write love poems.)*

Final Snarky Mic Drop:

You're not "giving up good food."

You're giving up blood sugar spikes, insulin tantrums, and afternoon death spirals.

You're not "on a diet."

You're **on a metabolic flex tour.**

Eat like someone who *finally* read the plot twist: The villain was bread the whole time.

CHAPTER 7:
EXERCISE — MOVE IT OR LOSE IT (TO INSULIN RESISTANCE)

You Don't Need a Gym Membership — Just a Pulse and a Playlist

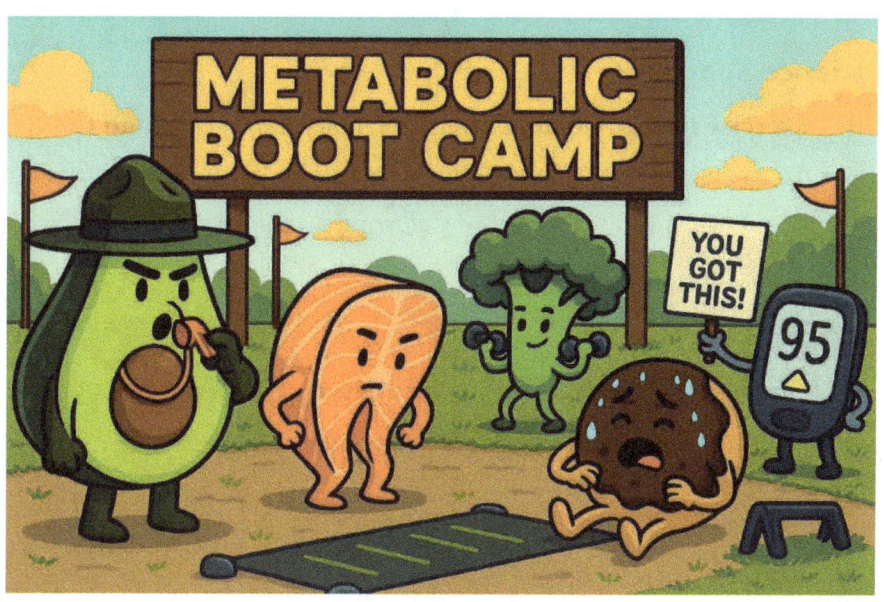

Let's clear this up right now: **Exercise is not punishment.** It's not penance for last year's birthday cake. It's not medieval torture for eating "off plan."

It's **a biochemical love letter** to your mitochondria.

You don't need to be a gym bro or a half-marathon Instagram martyr. You just need to **move**, consistently, **like your glucose depends on it**. (Spoiler: It does.)

Why Movement Is Your Glucose Cheat Code

Your muscles aren't just there for flexing selfies. They are **glucose sponges**. Biological black holes slurping up sugar **even WITHOUT insulin** — just because you moved them.

Translation: The more you move, the less your poor, overworked pancreas has to scream into the metabolic void.

Science Snapshot:

"Exercise improves insulin sensitivity by up to 40%, and the effect can last 24–72 hours post-activity."

— Colberg et al., Diabetes Care, 2016

Math Check:

- One 20-minute walk = up to three days of reduced glucose drama.
- ROI (Return on Insulin): Physiologic dividends paid in full.

START WHERE YOU ARE (Not Where #Fitspo Wants You To Be)

You don't need:

- A personal trainer named Brick (or Boulder or Tank).
- A gym selfie ring light (your kitchen lighting is just fine).
- Leggings that cost more than your grocery bill (spinach > spandex).

*You need **small, consistent wins**.*

Week	What to Do	Reality Check
Week 1	Walk 10 minutes after each meal	Pajamas = acceptable athletic wear.
Week 2	Add light dumbbells, resistance bands, bodyweight squats	Grunting encouraged, choreography optional.
Week 3+	Level up with yoga, planks, maybe an angry power walk	Looking silly burns more calories anyway.

Why Post-Meal Walks Are Bio-Hacks

- Muscles suck up glucose.
- Insulin sensitivity spikes.
- Post-meal blood sugar spikes get knee-capped.

"Walk after you eat" should be printed on every restaurant menu next to the dessert list.

Science Snapshot:

"Post-meal physical activity significantly blunts glucose excursions compared to remaining sedentary."
— *DiPietro et al., JAMA, 2013*

Translation: Your metabolism wants a walk, not a nap and an existential crisis. Mall laps: because aimless wandering is better than aimless insulin spikes. Grumbling about "kids these days" while speed-shuffling through your neighborhood? Medically encouraged.

How To Move Without Hating Yourself:

- **Kitchen Dance Battles:** *Burn carbs and your dignity. Worth it.*
- **Angry Power Walks:** Storm off imaginary arguments. Bonus calories if you add dramatic arm swings.
- **Aggressive Gardening:** Yard work = stealth metabolic rebellion.
- **Podcast Walks:** Nerd out while burning fat. It's multitasking, but make it rebellious.
- **Random Pushup Challenges:** Against the wall, the couch, your will to live. Doesn't matter. It counts.

Mini Workouts > Heroic Grand Gestures

- *10 minutes walking after meals.*
- *2 minutes of squats during streaming.*
- *1-minute planks while questioning your life choices.*

Consistency beats dramatic, unsustainable heroics every time.

Science Snapshot:

"Short bouts of moderate activity improve postprandial glucose control, independent of weight loss."

— Thorp et al., Diabetes Care, 2013

Translation: *You don't have to lose 50 pounds to start winning. You just have to get off the couch before your TV asks "Are you still watching?"*

Final Snarky Mic Drop:

Exercise is not punishment. *It's revenge. Revenge on insulin resistance. Revenge on inflammation. Revenge on every junk food marketing executive who lied to your face.*

EXERCISE

*You're not "working out." You're staging a **molecular-level coup d'état**.*

Move because you **respect your mitochondria**. Move because you **love your future self**. Move because sitting still is literally killing you — slowly and quietly.

CHAPTER 8:
GLUCOSE MONITORING —
THE FEEDBACK LOOP THAT SHAMES YOUR MEAL CHOICES

*Plot Twist — Your Oatmeal Is a Villain Wearing
a Blueberry Hat and a Maple Drizzle Mustache*

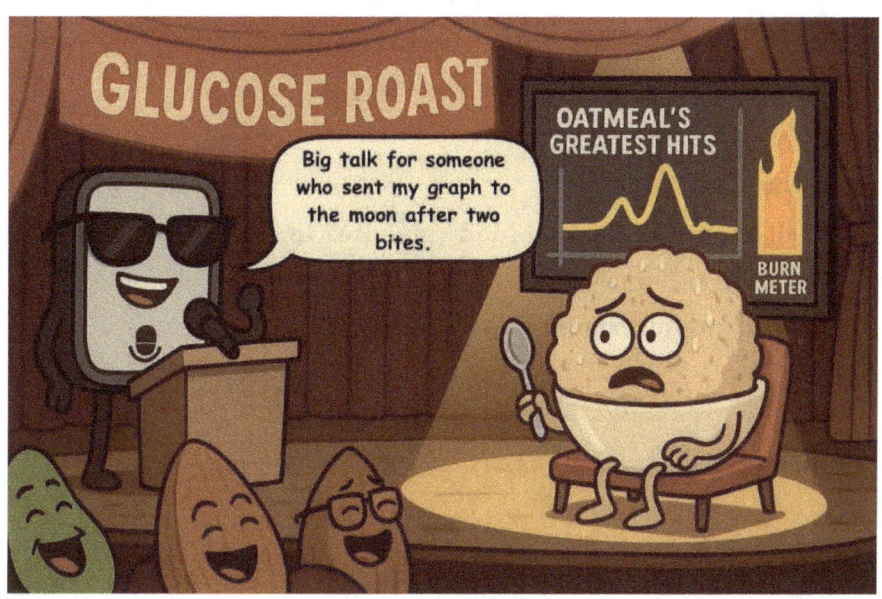

Welcome to the most awkward but life-saving part of your metabolic rebellion: **Glucose monitoring.**

You thought oatmeal was your friend? Your Continuous Glucose Monitor (CGM) is here to roast that lie harder than a stand-up comic with a glucose grudge.

If you're not measuring, you're guessing. And hope is not a reliable blood sugar strategy.

Why You Need To Test (Even If You Think You're "Eating Healthy")

- *CGMs and glucometers* **turn every meal into an experiment.**
- *You stop asking, "Is this healthy?"*
- *You start asking, "Is this healthy for me?"*

Because guess what? **Your metabolism isn't a democracy.** It's a biochemical dictatorship — and glucose monitors are the undercover agents leaking all the government secrets.

Science Snapshot:

"Self-monitoring of blood glucose improves glycemic control, enhances lifestyle modification, and accelerates patient empowerment."

— *American Diabetes Association, 2023*

Translation: *Data = power. Denial = diabetes' favorite wingman.*

When To Check Your Glucose:

Timing	Why It Matters
Fasting (morning)	See your baseline insulin drama.
Before meals	Know your starting line.
1–2 hours after meals	Catch the glucose explosion (or victory dance).
Before bed	Make sure your pancreas isn't throwing a rave overnight.

Golden Rule: You're not chasing perfection. You're hunting **clues** like a detective with a CGM strapped to your arm.

Blood Sugar Bullseye:

Type 2 Diabetes Glucose Targets: Ideal vs. ADA (American Diabetes Association) Standards

Situation	Metabolically Ideal	ADA Guidelines (2024)
Fasting	70–100 mg/dL	80–130 mg/dL
60-90 minutes post-meal	<120 mg/dL	<180 mg/dL (1–2 hrs post-meal)
2–3 hours post-meal	Back to baseline	Not specified

If your post-meal spike looks like the stock market right before a crash — Congratulations — you've just diagnosed your "healthy" food as metabolic sabotage. Nothing says "blood sugar control" like a glucose level that could caramelize a crème brûlée.

Science Snapshot:

> "Post-meal glucose levels above 120 mg/dL are linked to oxidative stress, inflammation, and vascular dysfunction—even in non-diabetics."
> — Ceriello et al., Diabetologia, 2008

Translation: Even a "healthy" spike can turn your bloodstream into a slow-motion biochemical crime scene. Bottom line: Your cells panic way before 180.

The Fix: Aim to keep post-meal glucose <120 mg/dL for optimal cellular serenity. Think of it as metabolic conflict prevention—because no one wants angry mitochondria plotting your downfall.

Tech That Tells The Brutal Truth:

Tool	Why It's Awesome
Dexcom G7 / Stelo	Live streaming your glucose sins in digital glory to your cell phone
Freestyle Libre 3 / Lingo	Your personal carb paparazzi—snapping every spike.
Glucose Buddy app	Graphs your food failures so you can laugh, cry, and learn.
MySugr app	Turns blood sugar logging into weirdly adorable cartoon avatar management.

Bonus Feature: Graphs that roast you *faster than a high school group chat.*

What You'll Learn (And Laugh About Later):

- *Your "healthy" oatmeal spikes glucose worse than actual cake.*
- *Walking for 10 minutes after eating can save your pancreas from sending out resignation letters.*
- *Stress and bad sleep jack up your glucose worse than binge-eating frosting directly from the tub.*
- And most importantly: You stop fearing food. You **start mastering** it.

Science Snapshot:

"Continuous glucose monitoring enhances behavioral modification, reduces glycemic variability, and promotes improved outcomes in Type 2 diabetes management."
— *Beck et al., JAMA, 2017*

Translation: Wearing a CGM is basically strapping a lie detector to your meals.

Final Snarky Mic Drop:

Glucose monitoring isn't about guilt. *It's about gathering **intel** like a metabolic Secret Agent. You're not punishing yourself. You're running a live-action science experiment where **the prize is your pancreas begging you for a thank-you card**.*

Data beats denial. Tracking beats guessing. Science beats shame. And yes, your oatmeal is still guilty.

PART III:
LEVELING UP YOUR COMEBACK STORY

CHAPTER 9:
SURVIVING REAL LIFE — CRAVINGS, PARTIES, AND PLATEAU PURGATORY

Blood Sugar vs. Birthday Cake — The Ultimate Boss Battle

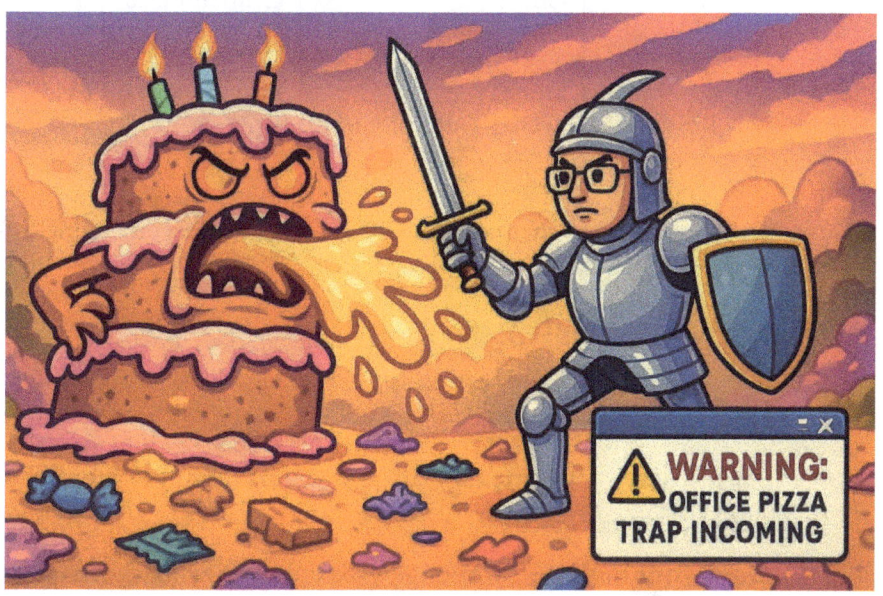

You've meal-prepped, grocery-mastered, glucose-monitored, and kitchen-overhauled like a biochemical rockstar. But now? **Real life enters the chat.** (And it brought donuts.)

Welcome to the **Metabolic Boss Level**: Cravings. Birthday parties. Office pizza ambushes. 11 PM existential crises powered by online rabbit holes and loneliness.

Congratulations — you're about to find out if your systems are strong or if cake still owns your soul.

Cravings: Attack Of The Snack Hormones

First, let's get scientific: **Cravings ≠ Hunger.** *Cravings are just your brain's lazy attempt to hack dopamine without doing any real emotional work.*

Situation	What Your Brain Craves	Why
Bored?	Cookies	Fake excitement.
Anxious?	Chips	Crunching as emotional therapy.
Tired?	Donuts	Fast glucose hit to fight sleep debt.

Translation: Cravings are chemical tantrums, not nutritional emergencies.

Craving Combat Strategies:

- ***Drink water first:*** *You're probably thirsty, not dying of Candy Bar Deficiency Syndrome.*
- **Eat protein + fat at meals:** Satiety murders cravings faster than willpower ever could.
- **Move your body:** A 10-minute walk shuts down snack-hunting brain circuits like a boss fight victory dance.
- **Delay, distract, delete:** Cravings are like drunk texts. Ignore them for 20 minutes — they lose their power and usually sound ridiculous afterward.

Surviving Social Landmines (Parties, Potlucks, And Betrayal Buffets)

It's Susan's birthday. The break room looks like a bakery exploded. Here's your tactical plan:

- **Pre-Game Your Insulin:** Eat a high-protein, high-fat meal *before* you go.
- **Bring a Decoy Dish:** Show up with a low-carb option so you don't end up in a glucose hostage situation.
- **Master the Polite Decline:** "That cake looks amazing, but my pancreas has trust issues." Smile. Sip your sparkling water. Move on like the metabolic ninja you are.
- **Fake Fullness If Necessary:** Hand on stomach, exaggerated sigh. It's dinner theater for your pancreas.

Science Snapshot:

"**Implementation intentions significantly reduce dietary lapses and improve self-regulatory success during high-risk situations.**"

— *Adriaanse et al., Health Psychology, 2011*

Translation: If you plan ahead, you win. If you show up hungry and unarmed, the ice cream cake wins.

Plateau Purgatory: Welcome To The Metabolic DMV

*You're doing everything right. You're logging meals, walking, sleeping like a melatonin-fueled sloth...and the scale **won't budge**.*

Cue the existential meltdown. Cue the questioning of all life choices. Cue the deep yearning to throw your CGM into the ocean.

Deep breath. Plateaus aren't failures. They are your metabolism chilling, recalibrating, preparing for the next boss fight.

You didn't break your body. You didn't "ruin" anything. You're not stuck. You're stabilizing.

How To Track Real Victories (When The Scale Is Misleading You)

Victory Type	Clues You're Winning
Blood sugar	Lower fasting glucose, fewer meal spikes
Mood	More stable, less hanger-induced rage
Sleep	Deeper, dreamier, less 3 AM existential crisis
Clothing	Waistbands that don't scream for mercy

Fun fact: Fat cells are drama queens. Sometimes they need time to pack up their emotional baggage before they leave.

Final Snarky Mic Drop:

One cookie doesn't end your rebellion. One stress binge isn't a personality flaw. One plateau isn't metabolic treason.

Log it. Laugh at it. Walk it off. (Literally.)

Your comeback isn't built on never falling. It's built on **getting up faster** — with sass, science, and a metaphorical baseball bat aimed at insulin resistance.

Consistency > Perfection.
Resilience > Restriction.
Laughing > Quitting.

Now put down the donut. You've got a rebellion to finish.

CHAPTER 10:
THIS ISN'T A DIET — IT'S A COMEBACK STORY

From Blood Sugar Train-wreck to A1c Zen

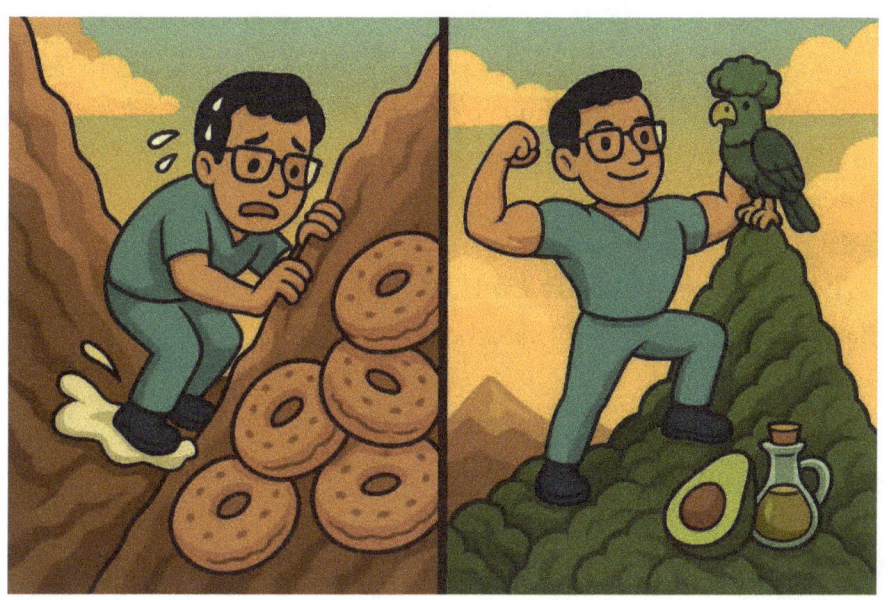

Let's rewind the glucose horror movie:

My A1c was 8.6%. My energy was somewhere between "sedated sloth" and "decomposing battery." My pants? Actively waging war against my dignity.

I wasn't living. I was glucose-surfing into metabolic oblivion.

Fast Forward: Ten Months Later

Metric	Before	After
A1c	8.6%	5.0%
Weight	+80 pounds	-80 pounds
Medications	0 started	0 needed
Energy	Sloth Mode	Toddler on Espresso
Food Guilt	Daily shame spirals	Replaced by data nerd smugness

No crash diets. No miserable celery-only purgatory. No expensive detox teas sold by influencers who can't spell "mitochondria." Just **science, systems, stubbornness, and strategic disrespect for the Standard American Diet.**

What Success Actually Looks Like:

Spoiler alert: It's not abs. It's not a kale smoothie selfie. It's THIS:

- Waking up *not* feeling like you've been hit by a truck.
- Eating meals without needing a web search to diagnose post-lunch regret.
- Fitting into jeans you had emotionally buried in 2008.
- Having a stable mood even when your coworker "accidentally" replies-all (again).

Metabolic Success isn't sexy. It's stubborn, boring consistency — and it feels better than any cheat day high.

Science Snapshot:

> "Intensive lifestyle interventions achieve diabetes remission in up to 60% of patients, with durability dependent on sustained weight loss and behavioral changes."
> — Lean et al., *The Lancet Diabetes & Endocrinology*, 2019

*Translation: This isn't magic. This isn't "lucky genetics." This is **basic biochemistry plus relentless rebellion**.*

From "Diet" To "Operating System":
You didn't "go on a diet." You installed a **new operating system**.

Less inflammation. Less insulin resistance. More mitochondria dancing awkwardly to smooth jazz in your cells.

This isn't about temporary suffering. This is about **permanent metabolic freedom**.

Mindset Upgrade Required:

Old Mindset	New Mindset
"I'm trying a diet."	"I'm building a system."
"I hope this works."	"I *engineer* my biochemistry now."
"I'll allow one cheat meal."	"I choose what fuels my rebellion."
"I have bad genetics."	"I have untapped mitochondrial rage."

New rule: You don't "cheat" anymore — you **strategize like a nerdy metabolic general**.

Final Snarky Mic Drop:
*You didn't just lose weight. You **evicted inflammation**. You **hijacked your glucose rollercoaster**. You **reprogrammed your mitochondria** like some kind of sarcastic, low-carb hacker. You're not managing diabetes. You're **rewriting the plot**. From metabolic hostage to glucose warlord. From hangry zombie to pancreas whisperer. From exhausted statistic to living, breathing, avocado-eating proof that **science wins**.*

CHAPTER 11:
MEDS, MYTHS, AND METABOLIC MIDDLEMEN

When to Take the Pill, Fire the Pill, or Roast the Pill Over a Bonfire

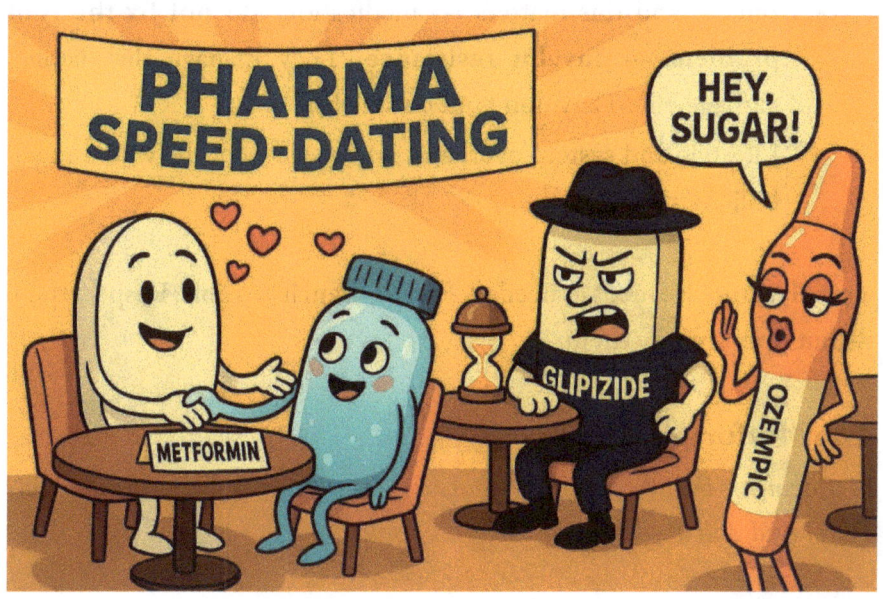

Let's talk about medications. Not with fear. Not with denial. With **science, sarcasm, and strategic intelligence**.

Because here's the truth:
- Meds aren't villains.
- Meds aren't saviors.
- Meds are TOOLS.

Sometimes you need a hammer. Sometimes you need a sledgehammer. Sometimes you just need to rebuild the whole damn house.

Know the difference — and don't let Big Pharma control your mitochondria.

Why Meds Exist (And Why They're Not A Life Sentence)
- *Type 2 diabetes is a spectrum, not a prison sentence.*
- Sometimes at diagnosis, your blood sugar is so astronomically wrecked that medications are life-saving, not optional.
- But — and this matters — medications **do not fix the root problem — Insulin resistance.** They manage the flaming garbage pile. They don't put out the fire.
- Lifestyle and system overhauls are what *reboot* the whole metabolic factory.

Translation: Use meds as needed. Escape them if possible. Respect them — but **don't marry them.**

The Metformin Memo
Metformin = the 80's pop star of diabetes drugs: Reliable, beloved, sometimes overplayed, still low-key iconic.

How It Works	Why Doctors Love It	Side Effects
Lowers liver's glucose production + increases insulin sensitivity	Cheap, effective, low side effect profile	Gastrointestinal chaos: gas, diarrhea, low-level regret

Pro Tip: If Metformin turns your gut into a protest zone - Ask for the extended-release. Take it with food. Blame it on modern pharmacology and move on.

Other Metabolic Characters You Might Meet:

Med Class	Nickname	Fun (or not) Facts
SGLT2 Inhibitors (Jardiance, Farxiga)	"Sugar Pee-ers"	Make you urinate glucose. Drink water or shrivel like a raisin.
GLP-1 Agonists (Ozempic, Mounjaro)	"Appetite Ninjas"	Crush hunger. Make celebrities whisper about you at brunch.
Sulfonylureas (Glipizide)	"Pancreas Pushers"	Squeeze insulin out aggressively. Sometimes too aggressively.
DPP-4 Inhibitors (Januvia)	"Quiet Interns"	Mild improvements. Won't set your house on fire, but won't rebuild it either.
Insulin	"The Big Gun"	Absolutely necessary sometimes. Sometimes a band-aid on a bread problem.

Science Snapshot:

> "Early intensive therapy of hyperglycemia improves beta-cell function and increases chances of remission."
> — Weng et al., NEJM, 2008

Translation: Sometimes meds are the short-term crutches **you need** *— so you can sprint later.*

But if your plan is "ride meds until they fail," spoiler alert: **They will.**

When To Rethink Your Meds (With Your Doctor — Not Social Media)

- A1c consistently under 6.0%.
- Post-meal glucose spikes barely making a ripple.
- No random overnight blood sugar raves.
- Lifestyle locked in tighter than Fort Knox.

Translation: Your body is acting like it has normal insulin sensitivity again.

Important: Never cowboy this alone. Your pancreas deserves a safe exit strategy, not a metabolic sneak attack.

What Meds Can (And Can't) Do:

Meds Can...	Meds Can't...
Buy time to fix root causes	Cure insulin resistance
Lower glucose temporarily	Replace muscle mass, sleep, or real food
Prevent short-term damage	Guarantee long-term reversal without lifestyle change

Wisdom: Use meds *strategically*. Build systems *permanently*.

Final Snarky Mic Drop:

*You are not a "failure" for needing meds. You are not a "hero" for avoiding meds. You are a **systems engineer** rebuilding your own metabolic empire. Take the crutches when you need them. Ditch them when you don't.*

And if Big Pharma thinks they can keep you on the hamster wheel forever? Tell them your mitochondria have entered their rebellion phase. (And that you brought science, sass, and salmon.)

CHAPTER 12:
RESOURCES FOR NERDS, NEWBIES, AND EVERYONE IN BETWEEN

Your Official Metabolic Toolbox — Science, Apps, and Snark Included

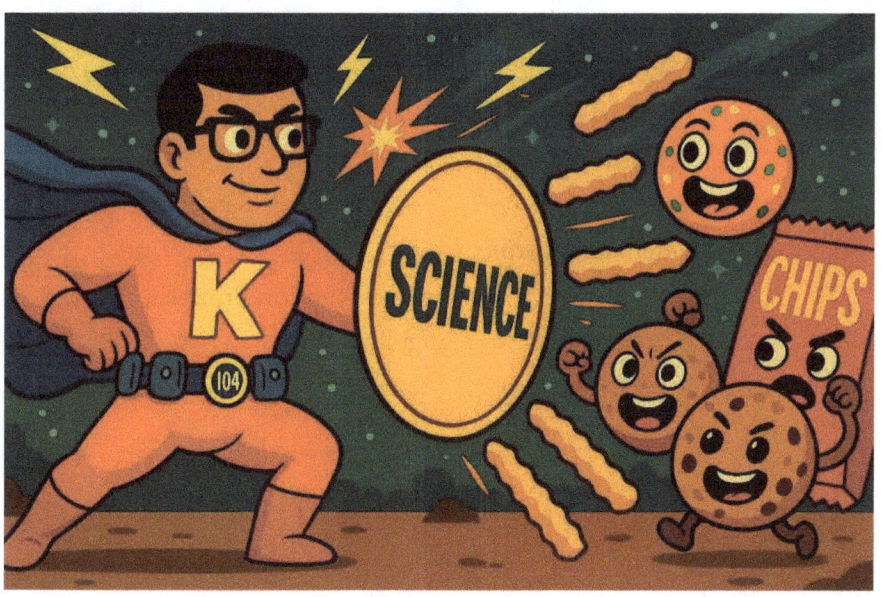

Congratulations, rebel. You've survived sarcasm, science, glucose graphs, and carb betrayal. **Now it's time to armor up** — because this isn't the end. It's just **leveling up**.

Here's your official Metabolic Survival Kit:
- Books.
- Apps.
- Communities.
- Gear.
- Enough nerd fuel to outsmart diabetes forever.

Communities: Because You're Not A Lone Wolf

- *Reddit:*
    - r/diabetes — Glucose chaos, memes, and brutal honesty.
    - r/ketogains — Where nerds and gym bros unite over metabolic rebellion.
- *Facebook Groups:*
    - "Reversing Type 2 Diabetes Support Group" — Empowering, science-based, and community-driven.
    - "Low-Carb Living" — Warning: Will contain 400 deviled egg recipes and emotional debates over cauliflower rice.
- *DiabetesDaily.com:* Forums, real stories, and occasional glucose gossip hotter than daytime TV.
- **Local Meetups:** YMCAs, libraries, support groups. (Yes, real humans exist offline. Shocking, I know.)
- **Bonus:** Some meetups offer free coffee. (Bring your own sarcasm.)

Apps That Turn You Into A Data Nerd (And Save Your Sanity)

App	Why You'll Love It
MyFitnessPal	Macro tracking without judgment (well...mostly).
CarbManager	Low carb macros + graphs = Spreadsheet joy.
Glucose Buddy	Your glucose journal that sometimes gently roasts you.
MySugr	Blood sugar logging disguised as a video game for adults.
Zero App	Intermittent fasting tracker — because discipline is easier with pretty graphs.

Pro Tip: If it makes you track, it makes you win.

Books That Won't Make You Launch Them Across The Room

The Diabetes Code — Dr. Jason Fung:
Why insulin, not calories, is your real nemesis.

Why We Get Sick — Dr. Ben Bikman:
Mitochondrial chaos, insulin resistance, and nerd-level empowerment.

Atomic Habits — James Clear:
The science of not relying on "motivation," ever again.

Metabolical — Dr. Robert Lustig:
A savage takedown of Big Food's decades-long misinformation campaign.

Eat Rich, Live Long — Ivor Cummins & Dr. Jeffry Gerber:
Hardcore low-carb science without cult weirdness.

Bonus:
All of these pair well with black coffee and mild rage at the traditional food pyramid.

Free Science Treasure Troves (Because You're A Nerd Now)

- *Virta Health Blog:* Clinical-grade diabetes reversal case studies (and tactical glucose mic drops).
- **Nutrition Coalition:** Holding outdated public nutrition policies accountable with spreadsheets and data.
- **DietDoctor.com:** Meal plans, low-carb guides, myth destruction...delivered with suspiciously calm Swedish precision.
- **American Diabetes Association (ADA):** Official guidelines (useful for arguing with insurance companies).

Gear For Metabolic Ninjas

- ***Continuous Glucose Monitor (CGM):*** *Dexcom, Libre, or anything that tattles on your glucose crimes in real-time.*
- **Food Scale:** Because "eyeballing" portions is how you accidentally eat six servings of almonds.
- **Cast Iron Skillet:** For steaks so righteous they might lower your glucose on sight.
- **Spiralizer:** Because real rebels turn zucchini into noodles instead of insulin spikes.
- **Good Walking Shoes:** Still the cheapest, most powerful blood-sugar-slaying tool on Earth.

Quotes To Staple To Your Fridge

- *"Data, not drama."*
- *"Progress, not perfection."*
- *"Every low-carb plate is a protest against insulin resistance."*
- *"Cravings are just thoughts — you don't have to RSVP."*
- *"If you're full, the ice cream can wait. Forever."*

Bonus Fridge Upgrade: Print a CGM graph of your worst food betrayal and hang it there. Motivational AND hilarious.

Final Mission Brief:

- ***Stay curious.*** *The science evolves — and so should you.*
- ***Stay consistent.*** Perfection is overrated. Consistency is undefeated.
- ***Stay laughing.*** Humor lowers cortisol. Cortisol raises glucose. Ergo: Laughing is medical therapy.

- ***Stay out of the bread aisle.*** Seriously. Just...trust me.
- ***Stay dangerous.*** Dangerous to sugar. Dangerous to excuses. Dangerous to insulin resistance.

You are not just surviving diabetes. You're engineering its retreat. With nerd weapons. With protein ammo. With science grenades. And with just enough sarcasm to keep it fun.

BONUS LEVEL

BONUS CHAPTER:
INTERMITTENT FASTING —
YOUR METABOLIC CHEAT CODE

How to Outsmart Your Insulin and Reboot Your Metabolism

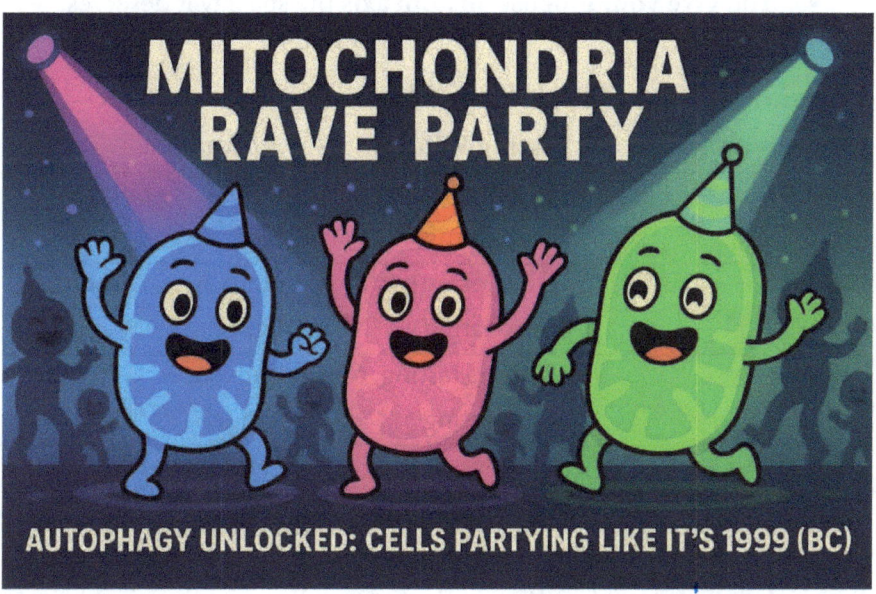

First things first:
- **Fasting is normal.**
- **Constant grazing is weird.**
- **You were biologically built for this.**

Our ancestors didn't have refrigerators or meal delivery services. Sometimes they fasted because the berry bush was empty and the local mammoth was really fast for its size.

Modern Translation: Fasting is a biological feature, not a design flaw.

What Intermittent Fasting (IF) Really Is:

*Think of it like **office hours for your pancreas**: Instead of working overtime 24/7 (and filing metabolic HR complaints), Insulin clocks in, does its job, clocks out, and finally gets to relax.*

- You **eat** during a set window.
- You **fast** the rest of the time.
- You **give your glucose-insulin axis** the spa day it deserves.

Popular IF Plans (Pick Your Flavor)

Style	Fasting Window	Nickname
12:12	12 hours fasting, 12 hours eating	"The Easy Entry Plan"
16:8	16 hours fasting, 8 hours eating	"Lunch-to-Dinner Club"
18:6	18 hours fasting, 6 hours eating	"Advanced Glucose Mode"
OMAD (One Meal a Day)	~23 hours fasting, 1-hour feast window	"Hardcore Hero"

Reminder: You don't have to win the fasting Olympics. You just have to give your metabolism a fighting chance.

Science Snapshot:

"Intermittent fasting improves insulin sensitivity, reduces oxidative stress, promotes autophagy, and enhances mitochondrial function."

— Longo et al., *Cell Metabolism*, 2019

Translation: Fasting makes your cells throw a microscopic rave with tiny mitochondrial party hats.

How Fasting Fixes The Metabolic Mess:

- *Lower Insulin:* Less poking the pancreas bear.
- *Stabilized Glucose:* No more "hangry" rollercoasters of doom.
- *Autophagy Activation:* Your cells clean like they're prepping for a metabolic open house.
- *Fat Burning:* Your body finally taps into those "emergency reserves" (aka the snack stash on your waistline).

Bonus: Mental clarity that feels suspiciously like upgrading your brain to first class from coach.

Common Fasting Myths (That Deserve To Be Set On Fire)

Myth	Reality
"Skipping breakfast ruins your metabolism!"	No, chronic overeating ruins it faster.
"You'll lose all your muscle!"	Only if you starve yourself, binge-watch reality shows, and forget protein exists.
"You need 6 small meals a day!"	That advice was sponsored by snack companies. Fight me.
"You'll faint from hunger!"	Hydration > Drama. Stay hydrated, stay upright.

Pro Tip: Hunger peaks and fades. It's a wave, not a death sentence.

How To Start Intermittent Fasting (Without Crying Or Screaming)

- *Start slow:* Stop eating at 7 PM. Don't eat until breakfast the next morning at 7 AM. (You don't need to go full monk on Day 1.)

- **Hydrate like a camel:** Water, black coffee, tea = friends. Milkshakes = betrayal.
- **Eat *real* meals when you eat:** When you feast, FEAST — protein, healthy fats, veggies. No sad rabbit food allowed.
- **Stay busy:** You're not "starving." You're just bored. Clean the garage. Call your weird uncle. Go fight capitalism.
- **Celebrate small wins:** Each hour you fast is a metabolic flex.

FASTING FAQS: Quick-Fire Round

Question	Answer
Coffee during fasting?	YES — black or unsweetened tea, too.
Exercise while fasting?	YES — burn fat, not tears.
Will I pass out?	Only if dehydrated, sleep-deprived, or dramatically overacting.
Should everyone fast?	NO — talk to a doctor if you're pregnant, underweight, or fighting eating disorders.

Real Talk: My Fasting Wins (That Weren't In The Brochures)

- *No more mid-morning snack panic.*
- *Insulin sensitivity boosted like a space rocket.*
- *Mental clarity that made me question my previous life choices.*
- *Energy better than any overpriced green juice promised me.*

Side Effect: Wearing smug facial expressions around carb addicts. (100% unavoidable.)

Final Snarky Mic Drop:

*Fasting isn't about suffering. It's about **liberating your mitochondria** from the biochemical daycare that is constant snacking.*

You're not starving. You're **retraining your metabolism**. You're **reclaiming metabolic flexibility**. You're **rewriting the manual on how your body runs energy ops**. You're not dieting. You're evolving. And evolution is hungry for rebels.

CONCLUSION:
WELCOME TO THE REST OF YOUR LIFE

This Isn't the End. It's the Origin Story.

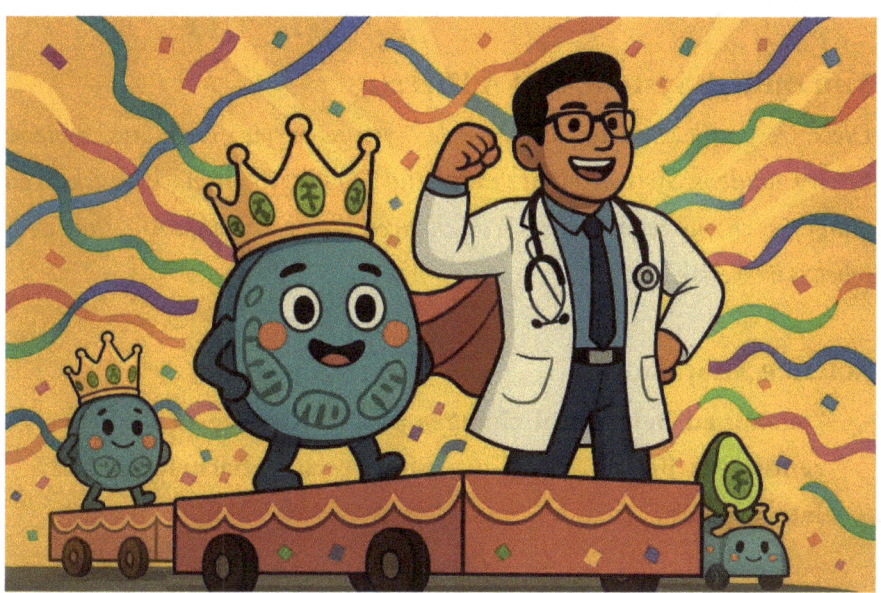

You didn't just read a book. You engineered a metabolic jailbreak. You rewired your mitochondria. You filed divorce papers against the Standard American Diet. You took your pancreas out of witness protection.

You rebelled. Against bad science. Against broken systems. Against every cereal aisle that whispered lies to your blood sugar for decades. **And you won.**

Let's Recap Your Metabolic Glow-Up:
- *Fired your broken fuel system (sugar).*
- *Rehired the one that actually works (fat + muscle + science).*

- *Demolished insulin resistance with grocery carts, not guilt trips.*
- *Weaponized walking, fasting, and data like a nerdy health assassin.*
- *Ate real food without channeling the energy of someone who just lost a fight with a buffet.*
- *Turned glucose monitoring into a biochemical smackdown instead of a shame spiral.*

You Built A System, Not A Diet:

Diets are fragile. Systems are durable. Systems survive birthdays. Systems survive holidays. Systems survive existential Tuesday night snack attacks. You didn't just change what you ate. You changed **how you think***. And that, dear rebel, is irreversible.*

Science Snapshot:

> **"Sustained behavioral changes predict long-term diabetes remission better than any short-term pharmacological intervention."**
>
> — Wing et al., Diabetes Care, 2021

Translation: *You didn't need another medication. You needed a system upgrade. And you just installed it.*

Final Life Commandments: Tattoo Them On Your Brain (Maybe)

- *Consistency beats motivation.*
- *Walking is still undefeated.*
- *Blood sugar doesn't lie, but marketing usually does.*
- *Eat like your mitochondria have feelings. (Because they do.)*
- *Laugh at failures. Track wins. Keep moving.*

Final Final Snarky Mic Drop:

You are not a number on a scale. You are not an A1c value. You are not a health insurance diagnosis code. You are **a biochemical rebellion in progress**.

You're the proof that chronic disease doesn't get the final word. You're the reminder that science, humor, stubbornness, and steak can rewrite destiny.

You didn't just survive. You **started a rebellion**. And it's only getting louder.

Welcome To The Rest Of Your Life:

Fueled by fiber. Powered by protein. Armored by muscle. Backed by relentless science. Laughed through every failure, because you're just that stubborn.

The system is yours now. Welcome home, rebel.

Now go eat some protein, lift something heavy, laugh too loud, and make insulin resistance cry in a corner like you own it…because you do.

Khalid Saeed, D.O.
Physician | Patient | Glucose Whisperer

ABOUT THE AUTHOR

Dr. Khalid Saeed, D.O. *is a board-certified physician who learned the hard way that diagnosing diabetes is a lot easier than living with it. After years of prescribing lifestyle changes with one hand while mindlessly eating granola bars with the other, Dr. Saeed had his metabolic wake-up call with his own Type 2 diabetes diagnosis.*

Rather than surrendering to meds and memes about quinoa cleanse bowls, he launched a full-scale rebellion—powered by PubMed, stubbornness, sarcasm, and an unreasonable amount of roasted Brussels sprouts. Ten months later, he reversed his diabetes, reclaimed his health, and became living proof that: Science works. Systems matter. Humor heals.

When he's not battling insulin resistance like a nerdy superhero, he can be found flying small planes in a love-hate relationship with gravity, creating low-carb recipes with unnecessarily dramatic names, debating if lettuce counts as an emotional support vegetable, and proving that science, snark, and spinach can, in fact, coexist.

You can reach Dr. Saeed at TampaBayConciergeDoctor.com or on Instagram @dr.khalid.saeed

REFERENCES

(For the science nerds who want receipts.)

Adriaanse, M. A., de Ridder, D. T. D., & de Wit, J. B. F. (2011). Implementing intentions to eat healthily: Crucial aspects and relevant processes. Health Psychology Review, 5(1), 10–25.

American Diabetes Association. (2023). Standards of medical care in diabetes—2023. Diabetes Care, 46(Supplement_1), S1–S291.

Beck, R. W., Riddlesworth, T. D., Ruedy, K., Ahmann, A., Bergenstal, R. M., Haller, S., ... & Price, D. (2017). Effect of continuous glucose monitoring on glycemic control in adults with Type 1 diabetes using insulin injections: The DIAMOND randomized clinical trial. JAMA, 317(4), 371–378.

Colberg, S. R., Sigal, R. J., Fernhall, B., Regensteiner, J. G., Blissmer, B. J., Rubin, R. R., ... & Braun, B. (2016). Exercise and Type 2 diabetes: The American College of Sports Medicine and the American Diabetes Association joint position statement. Diabetes Care, 39(11), 2065–2079.

Ceriello, A., Esposito, K., Piconi, L., Ihnat, M. A., Thorpe, J. E., Testa, R., & Giugliano, D. (2008). Oscillating glucose is more deleterious to endothelial function and oxidative stress than mean glucose in normal and Type 2 diabetic patients. Diabetologia, 51(10), 1838–1841.

DiPietro, L., Gribok, A., Stevens, M. S., Hamm, L. F., & Rumpler, W. V. (2013). Three hours of prolonged sitting reduces postprandial glucose metabolism in healthy older adults. The Journals of Gerontology: Series A, 68(7), 769–775.

Gorin, A. A., Wing, R. R., Fava, J. L., Jakicic, J. M., & Jeffery, R. (2005). Weight loss treatment influences untreated spouses and the home environment: Evidence of a ripple effect. International Journal of Obesity, 29(10), 1235–1242.

Gudzune, K. A., Welsh, C., Lane, E., Choi, T., & Appel, L. J. (2015). The impact of financial incentives on weight loss and weight loss maintenance: A systematic review. Obesity (Silver Spring), 23(9), 1780–1789.

Hall, K. D., Kahan, S., & Westman, E. C. (2019). Low-carbohydrate diets for the treatment of obesity and Type 2 diabetes: A systematic review and meta-analysis. Nutrition Reviews, 77(5), 326–337.

Jakubowicz, D., Barnea, M., Wainstein, J., & Froy, O. (2013). High caloric intake at breakfast vs. dinner differentially influences weight loss and glycemic control in obese individuals. Obesity, 21(12), 2504–2512.

Lean, M. E. J., Leslie, W. S., Barnes, A. C., Brosnahan, N., Thom, G., McCombie, L., ... & Taylor, R. (2019). Durability of a primary care–led weight-management intervention for remission of Type 2 diabetes: 2-year results of the DiRECT open-label, cluster-randomised trial. The Lancet Diabetes & Endocrinology, 7(5), 344–355.

Longo, V. D., Panda, S., & Mattson, M. P. (2019). Fasting: Molecular mechanisms and clinical applications. Cell Metabolism, 29(3), 427–446.

Ludwig, D. S., Majzoub, J. A., Al-Zahrani, A., Dallal, G. E., Blanco, I., & Roberts, S. B. (2002). High glycemic index foods, overeating, and obesity. JAMA, 287(18), 2414–2423.

Saslow, L. R., Mason, A. E., Kim, S., Goldman, V., Ploutz-Snyder, R., Bayandorian, H., ... & Moran, P. J. (2017). An online intervention comparing a very low-carbohydrate ketogenic diet and lifestyle recommendations versus a plate method diet in overweight individuals with Type 2 diabetes: A randomized controlled trial. Nutrition & Diabetes, 7(12), e256.

Taylor, R., Al-Mrabeh, A., Zhyzhneuskaya, S., Peters, C., Barnes, A. C., Aribisala, B. S., ... & Holman, R. R. (2012). Remission of human Type 2 diabetes requires decrease in liver and pancreas fat content but is independent of weight loss. Diabetologia, 55(10), 2552–2563.

Weng, J., Li, Y., Xu, W., Shi, L., Zhang, Q., Zhu, D., ... & Yan, X. (2008). Effect of intensive insulin therapy on β-cell function and glycemic control in newly diagnosed Type 2 diabetes: A multicentre randomised parallel-group trial. The New England Journal of Medicine, 361(9), 867–876.

Wing, R. R., Tate, D. F., Gorin, A. A., Raynor, H. A., & Fava, J. L. (2006). A self-regulation program for maintenance of weight loss. The New England Journal of Medicine, 355(15), 1563–1571.

SUGGESTED READING

(For Metabolic Nerds, Glucose Rebels, and Curious Humans)

Want to dive deeper into the science (and sass) behind kicking Type 2 diabetes to the curb?

Here's a curated list of books, blogs, and resources that helped sharpen my rebellion — and might supercharge yours too.

Must-Read Books

The Diabetes Code — *Dr. Jason Fung*
How insulin resistance really works, why calories aren't the full story, and how intermittent fasting can reboot your metabolism.

Why We Get Sick — *Dr. Ben Bikman*
A nerdy deep-dive into how insulin resistance links to almost every chronic disease you're trying to avoid. Bonus: mitochondrial empowerment.

Atomic Habits — *James Clear*
Because beating Type 2 diabetes isn't about motivation — It's about tiny, relentless systems that quietly win the war.

Metabolical — *Dr. Robert Lustig*
A full-throttle takedown of processed food, Big Sugar, and metabolic mayhem. (Warning: may induce grocery store rage.)

Eat Rich, Live Long — *Ivor Cummins & Dr. Jeffry Gerber*
Low-carb science, myth-busting, and real-world advice — without the cult-like weirdness.

Favorite Nerdy Blogs and Websites

Virta Health Blog —
Clinical-grade articles on diabetes reversal, metabolic health, and why you don't need to fear fat.
virtahealth.com/blog

DietDoctor.com —
Low-carb, keto, fasting guides, recipe libraries, and myth-busting videos — delivered with calming Swedish precision.
dietdoctor.com

Nutrition Coalition —
Science-first nutrition advocacy that fights back against decades of dietary dogma.
nutritioncoalition.us

DiabetesDaily.com —
Forums, stories, tools, and the occasional glucose gossip you didn't know you needed.
diabetesdaily.com

Tools That Helped Me Stop Guessing

- **Dexcom G7 (Stelo) / Freestyle Libre 3 (Lingo)** — Continuous glucose monitors that turn your body into a real-time glucose science project.
- **MyFitnessPal** — If you want a casual relationship with your macros (not an obsessive one).

- **CarbManager** — Low-carb macros, visual graphs, and keto cult energy — use wisely.
- **Zero App** — For tracking fasting windows and heroic acts of coffee-fueled willpower.

Final Thought

Reading is good. Applying what you read — even in tiny, imperfect, hilariously messy ways — is **better**. Knowledge without action is just trivia. Knowledge + rebellion = metabolic freedom. Now go forth and out-nerd your pancreas.

GLOSSARY OF TERMS

A1c (Hemoglobin A1c) - A lab test showing your average blood sugar over the past 2–3 months. Think of it as a metabolic report card.

ADA (American Diabetes Association) - The OG of diabetes guidelines. They've done more for awareness than anyone—but let's just say our glucometers sometimes disagree.

Autophagy - Cellular self-cleaning service where your body recycles damaged parts — boosted during fasting.

Beta Cells - The pancreas's insulin-producing rockstars (or exhausted interns if you have Type 2 diabetes).

Blood Glucose (Blood Sugar) - The concentration of sugar circulating in your bloodstream, aka metabolic rocket fuel or potential disaster zone.

CGM (Continuous Glucose Monitor) - A tiny wearable device that tattles on your real-time glucose sins — in glorious 24/7 graphs.

Cravings - False alarms sent by your brain demanding sugar for reasons like boredom, anxiety, or streaming-induced existentialism.

Cytokines - Tiny molecular messengers that your immune system fires off like frantic text messages — sometimes saving your life, sometimes starting drama (think inflammation, autoimmune chaos, or a full-body temper tantrum).

Dawn Phenomenon - An early morning hormone surge (cortisol, growth hormone) that tells your liver to dump glucose—just when your cells are least ready for it. Result: rising blood sugar before breakfast, no pancakes required.

Diabetes Remission (Reversal) - When Type 2 diabetes blood sugars return to a non-diabetic range without (or with minimal) medication, driven by major lifestyle changes—not magic.

Glycemic Index (GI) - A ranking of foods based on how fast they spike your blood sugar — spoiler: oatmeal is not innocent.

Gluconeogenesis - The emergency backup plan where your liver biohacks new sugar out of random parts like protein and fat — because apparently, we can't be trusted to eat carbs responsibly.

Glucometer- A handheld device that checks your blood sugar. The metabolic truth-o-meter.

Hyperinsulinemia - When your pancreas floods your bloodstream with insulin like it's frantically trying to silence a glucose riot — a sign of insulin resistance.

Insulin - The hormone that unlocks your cells so glucose can enter. When it's ignored, chaos ensues.

Insulin Resistance - When your cells ghost insulin harder than your worst blind date, leading to higher blood sugar.

Intermittent Fasting (IF) - An eating schedule that lets your insulin levels chill out, burn fat, and throw tiny mitochondrial parties.

Glossary of Terms

Keto Diet - A low-carb, high-fat eating style that turns your body into a fat-burning machine — not to be confused with a butter-worshipping cult.

Low-Carb Diet - An eating approach that reduces carbohydrate intake to lower insulin demands and stabilize glucose, with olive oil and avocados starring as heroes.

Metabolic Flexibility - Your body's ability to efficiently switch between burning carbs and fat for energy — a skill you probably lost somewhere between snack times.

Mitochondria - The microscopic power plants in your cells. Abuse them and you feel like garbage. Feed them right and you turn into a glucose-slaying superhero.

Net Carbs - Marketing math magic subtracting fiber and sugar alcohols from total carbs to make snack bars seem innocent. Proceed with caution.

Postprandial Glucose - Blood sugar levels after a meal. Ideally not resembling a stock market crash.

Protein + Fiber + Fat (PFF) - The "The Snack-Prevention Task Force" — eating these together keeps you full, happy, and less likely to fistfight a vending machine.

Standard American Diet (SAD) - An unfortunate acronym for a high-carb, high-sugar, processed-food-heavy eating pattern responsible for a lot of metabolic misery.

Visceral Fat - The dangerous fat around your organs whispering mean things to your pancreas and fueling chronic inflammation.

www.ingramcontent.com/pod-product-compliance
Lightning Source LLC
Chambersburg PA
CBHW070528030426
42337CB00016B/2149